The Diabetes Office Visit

The Diabetes Office Visit

*Helping You
Help Your Doctor
Help You*

David Calder, MD

David Calder Publishing
Creswell, Oregon

Drawing and picture on cover by Dr. Calder
Design by Sherry Green
Text set in Minion Pro, 11pt
Title set in News Gothic Std.

Printed in the United States of America

10 9 8 7 6 5 4 3 2 1   09 10 11 12 13 14 15 16 17 18 19

ISBN: 978-1-4563-1788-1

To my patients—
who taught me so much about life, the value of
persistence and kindness, and the quality of being
generally tough when it comes down to things that
really matter.

Contents

Contents continued

Acknowledgments

Writing this is difficult for me because I have had the pleasure of working with so many dedicated, special people, and the page is not long enough to list everyone. I will always remember the fun that Jeanne Johnston RN CDE, Jodie Donnely RD CDE, Julie Scalisi RD CDE, Darlene Hill, and I had developing the Diabetes Wellness Center. I also appreciate the support from Jan Smulovitz MD. We and our patients experienced the benefits of a team effort with diabetes management. In 1995 we joined PeaceHealth Medical Group and had the pleasure of working with Ida Martin RN CDE, Vicki Stave RD CDE, Kathleen Brandt RD CDE, David Hascall RN CDE, and a number of other dietitians. John Nelson PA CDE joined us a few years later. The other physicians in the Diabetes, Endocrine & Metabolism Service included Byron Musa MD, Jane Farmer MD, Matt Davies MD PhD, John Bagdade MD, and Ron Cirullo MD PhD. All contributed and made the diabetes program work.

I would like to further acknowledge Sacred Heart Medical Center in Eugene, Oregon for the high quality of care they provide for our community. I had always just taken this for granted until my wife, Marilyn, became critically ill and was in the Four

South ICU for two months. I was able to observe the amazing medical skills of my fellow physicians and nurses blended with the kindness and caring of everyone involved in her care. I believe it was that special blend of fantastic skills with kindness and caring from the heart that has allowed my wife and me to continue our life's journey together.

I would like to give special thanks to my daughter Lori Miller RN, owner of BrightStar Healthcare in Portland, Oregon, who suggested and then pushed me to write this book.

Doctor Calder's Biography

David Calder, MD, received his Bachelor of Science degree from Texas A & M University and his Doctor of Medicine degree from University of Texas Southwestern Medical School. He interned at San Joaquin General Hospital near Stockton, California, where he served his internal medicine residency, achieving Chief Resident in the third year. Dr. Calder was awarded a Diabetes and Metabolism fellowship at the University of Oregon Medical School Hospitals and Clinics in Portland, Oregon. He practiced diabetes and internal medicine in Eugene, Oregon, for thirty-five plus years. There, he was the cofounder of the Lane County Diabetes Association and the Director of the Diabetes Wellness Center, and served as a diabetes consultant for the Oregon Research Institute. Then in 1996 he and his associates, Byron Musa MD and Jane Farmer MD, and the Diabetes Wellness Center staff joined PeaceHealth Medical Group in Eugene Oregon as part of the Diabetes Endocrine and Metabolism Service. As a physician in this group he, along with John Bagdade MD, was instrumental in launching the Diabetes Wellness Assessment Program (DWAP) in PeaceHealth Clinics in Oregon, Washington, and Alaska.

Of his family life, Dr. Calder says, "I have got to be one of the luckiest guys around to have been blessed with my wife Marilyn, my children Julie (Radostitz), Lori (Miller), and Paul; my son-in-law Vince, daughter-in-law Brenda, and ex son-in-law Tim; and my grandchildren Halie, Brennen, Lucas, Mia, and Gretchen. What a deal. Life is good.

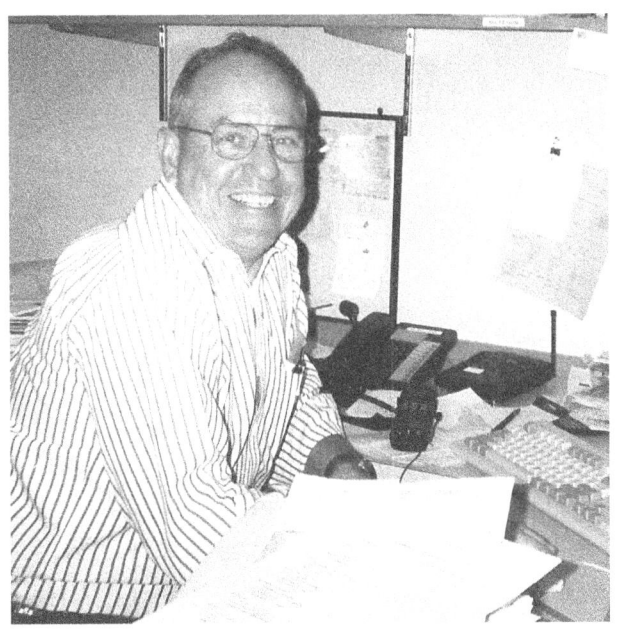

A Message to You—

The information discussed in this book, including my opinions, is for educational use only. My goal is to improve diabetes management discussions between you and your diabetes care provider. Do not change or adjust any medication without your physician's approval. Diabetes management is very personal, and decisions are based on your specific situation. Any decisions about insulin, diabetes oral medications, or blood sugar testing should be between you and your physician.

—David Calder, MD

Introduction
Greyhound vs. Hertz Car Rental

So, you have *diabetes mellitus*; too bad, there are no guaranties in life. There are opportunities, however, and you have been given the opportunity to work hard to preserve and maintain your good health. You could not have picked a better time in history to have this disease. There are amazing medications and technical skills available to help you manage diabetes mellitus and prevent its damaging effects on your body.

The gateways to this information are your doctor, diabetes educators, dietitians, and other health care personnel. So how do you as a patient get through the gate to reach this storehouse of information? I believe it starts with the office visit.

Your visit with the doctor may be the most difficult, time-consuming visit your doctor will have that day—your preparation and approach to that visit will determine the outcome. This book can serve as your guide to a successful visit.

A few years ago I heard a doctor explain that there are two types of office visits, "the Greyhound and the Hertz Car Rental style visits." Some of you may recall the Greyhound bus advertisement that went something like this: "Sit back, relax, and leave the driving to us." The Hertz Car Rental advertisement was, as I recall, "Let us put you in the driver's seat." The Greyhound approach will work for most office visits, but it does not work for a person with diabetes. Why is a diabetes visit so different? I believe it is because more than ninety-five percent of diabetes management is done by you, the patient, and not by your doctor.

This book is about slipping you into the driver's seat and using your doctor as the wise navigator to help you chart a course to a little place called Good Health. There will be some ups and downs and maybe a detour or two in trying to find this place, but it is there.

Have a safe trip!

Chapter 1

Two Devils – The Lows and the Highs

People with diabetes mellitus may often feel that they are caught between two devils: the devil of low and the devil of high blood glucose levels.

The Devil of Lows

The devil of low glucose can have an immediate impact on a person's life, with shaking, sweating, anxiety, and often confusion. This can progress to poor decision-making and even to loss of consciousness. This is very real and may lead to more serious problems such as falls and automobile accidents. This devil may be sneaky and will not always provide the early warning signals of shakiness or trembling, sweating, and anxiety, instead starting with confusion and difficulty in thinking, and then progressing to unconsciousness or even seizures. This devil is quick and dangerous and may strike more often the closer you get to normal glucose levels and when A1c results are less than 7. I have found that some medications cause more of a problem than others. I most often saw low blood glucose levels in the middle of the night with NPH insulins or combinations of NPH and rapid-acting insulins taken at dinnertime. Morning NPH (Neutral Protamine Hagedorn) insulin is often associated with low afternoon glucose levels. All sulfonylurea drugs can cause problems, but I personally saw more problems with glyburide and glimepiride. Low blood glucose levels associated with sulfonylurea drugs can last for days and may require hospitalization for treatment. This devil has some enablers that magnify the problem, the most common of which are inconsistent intake of carbohydrate, older age, and impaired kidney function.

Older age is also associated with loss of muscle mass, which may cause difficulty with interpretation of commonly used kidney tests. They may appear better than they actually are, especially serum creatinine levels.

I, personally, have had the least amount of problems with Lantus insulin, metformin (Glucophage), exenatide (Byetta), and pioglitazone (Actos), and I tried to avoid the use of NPH insulin and sulfonylurea drugs, especially in older people.

Why use something that may cause a problem if you don't have to? NPH insulin has a peak effect six to eight hours after it is taken. This means that NPH insulin taken at dinnertime is going to have its strongest effect between 1:00 AM and 3:00 AM. This is a time when we are all the most vulnerable to having low blood glucose levels. Talk to your doctor if you are having low blood glucose problems, and look for other choices in your treatment plan. The take-home message is to avoid NPH insulin at dinnertime, if possible.

The Devil of Highs

The devil of high sugars is always sneaky and usually silent. This devil takes years to do its devastating damage to your eyes, kidneys, nerves, and cardiovascular system. This devil may also travel with equally dangerous silent partners.

These silent partners will focus their attacks on your blood vessels. Ultimately, they may cause amputations, heart disease, and strokes for people with diabetes mellitus. These silent partners include "The Smoker" and other friends.

- Elevated blood pressure >130/80

- Mild kidney damage–albumin/creatinine ratio >30

- Cholesterol >200

- LDL cholesterol >70

- HDL cholesterol = men <40, women <50

- Triglycerides >150

•••

The goal of this book is to help you navigate a path between these two devils and avoid the disruption they can cause in your life. I warn you that this path is neither perfect nor easy. It has many potholes, curves, ups and downs, and dark corners, but it is still passable.

Just do your best.

As I look back over my thirty-five plus years of helping people manage this disease with imperfect tools, I can say that most people who did their best to achieve the existing goals available to them did not have to endure the severe complications of this disease. They were able to live long, healthy, active, productive lives.

Chapter 2
Setting Goals and Talking to Your Doctor

Y ou are in the driver's seat. A visit with your doctor is a business meeting; you are paying for your doctor's expert advice and counsel on how to manage your diabetes. Please remember that managing diabetes is more than just taking care of blood glucose levels. Your job includes all of the other risk factors associated with this disease.

Here are a few suggestions for planning your visit:

1. If you do not have current results of the tests listed on the goal sheet given below, contact your doctor's office and request that tests are done before your next visit. Be sure to have a copy of the results sent to you. The A1c (number 2 on the goal sheet at the end of this chapter) is recommended every three months, and the other laboratory tests (numbers 3–8 on the goal sheet) can be done a minimum of one time each year. Record the results in the "Your Results" column on the goal sheet. Now schedule your visit.

2. Schedule a visit specifically to discuss your lab results and to set goals.

3. Remember that you scheduled a business meeting. You have about five minutes to make your case. Don't waste time. Be precise and clear about what you want. You are in charge. Explain to your doctor that you are setting goals for your diabetes management and that you want his or her advice in the process. Show your goal sheet. After you agree on the target goals, ask, "Can you help me reach these goals?"

If the answer is yes, pick one or two goals to work on, ask for advice on how to reach your target, then schedule a follow-up visit to discuss your progress. I recommend two to three weeks for the next visit. Keep this process going until you have worked your way through all of your goals.

If the answer to "Can you help me reach these goals?" is no, ask for a referral to someone who *can* help your reach your goals.

It is just that easy. Now go do it. Remember that you are in charge of your health management. Your goal is to stay healthy and avoid the complications of this disease. It is up to you to reach those targets. Since you are in charge, it is also your responsibility to record and keep track of your results and to have them with you for each visit to your doctor.

Congratulations, you are now an active participant in managing this disease.

Goal Sheet
(Decide on your goals after discussion with your physician)

Test	Suggested Goal	Your Results	Your Goal
1. Home blood sugar test			
Before breakfast	90 to 130		
Before lunch	90 to 130		
Before dinner	90 to 130		
Before bedtime	100 to 140		
3:00 AM	90 to 130		
2. A1c hemoglobin	7		
3. Blood pressure (BP)	130/80		
4. Albumin/creatinine ratio	<30		
5. Cholesterol total	<200		
6. LDL cholesterol	<70		
7. HDL cholesterol			
In men	>40		
In women	>50		
8. Triglyceride	<150		
9. Abdominal girth			
For males	<40 inches		
For females	<35 inches		
10. Foot exam (yearly)			
11. Eye exam (yearly)			

Chapter 3

Home Blood Sugar Testing – Routine and Diagnostic Programs

When to test? How often to test? When do I need a full-court press? Here are a few of my ideas and guidelines to consider: blood sugar testing, and the recording of results thereof, is expensive, time-consuming, slightly uncomfortable, and always inconvenient. You have other tools to help you control your blood sugar that are equally inconvenient but less expensive. When do I use all or some of these tools?

The Tools

1. Blood sugar testing and the recording of results in a useful fashion

2. Diet records estimating and recording your carbohydrate intake

3. Exercise records

4. Medication records

When to use just one or all of your tools is the question. I would suggest you have a Routine Monitoring Program and a Diagnostic Program. Your routine program may vary depending on your diabetes medications.

Routine Monitoring Program

➤**If your A1c test is within your target goals and you are taking oral diabetes medication:**

- Test before breakfast daily

- Test before one of your other meals or at bedtime daily. Vary this test daily if possible. (Test before lunch one day and before dinner or at bedtime the next day.) If you are not ill and have an occasional blood sugar test not within your target range, this is often a food-related issue and will correct itself. I would suggest testing your blood before your next meal or bedtime. If it remains elevated switch to a Diagnostic Program.

➤**If you are taking oral diabetes medication plus Lantus or Levemir Insulin or bedtime NPH insulin:**

Lantus and bedtime NPH insulins are used to control your before-breakfast blood glucose. You can be trained to adjust these insulins to control your before-breakfast blood glucose in order to meet your goals. I prefer to use Lantus insulin for this purpose, as I believe that Lantus insulin has a lower risk of low blood sugars and provides a stable, non-peaking baseline insulin for twenty-four hours.

➤**If you require multiple insulin injections or insulin pumps:**

Your recommended routine testing is four times a day or more. Testing before meals and bedtime with an occasional 3:00 AM test is a good idea. Learn how to adjust insulin based on your home blood sugar test results.

Diagnostic Program

1. Test blood sugars before meals and at bedtime

2. Record blood sugar results

3. Keep food records

4. Review diabetes medication and ask yourself a few questions:

   •Did I miss a shot or a pill?

   •Is my insulin outdated?

   •Did I make a mistake?

   •Is the dose correct?

5. Have there been any recent changes in my exercise routine?

6. Am I coming down with an illness? Unexplained increases in your blood glucose may occur very early in a developing infection. Asymptomatic urinary tract infections in older women are a common cause for unexplained blood glucose elevations. One helpful hint of infection is a fairly uniform increase in all of the before-meal glucose results. Wide swings in the before-meal glucose test suggest erratic carbohydrate intake. (Oops! I just gave away one of my diagnostic skills. Oh well; you seem like a nice person. Just do not ask me to define *older women*.)

If the situation corrects itself, return to your routine testing. **If it does not correct itself, or if you are ill, contact your physician's office.** Be sure to bring your testing and food records with you for the visit.

Uncontrolled Diabetes

If your A1c hemoglobin is out of your target range, your blood sugar tests are out of your target range, in which case I suggest staying in the Diagnostic Program and working with your physician until the problems are corrected.

Chapter 4

Record Keeping – For You and Your Physician

Keeping Accurate Blood Glucose and Diet Records

This is one of the most difficult—and one of the most important—tasks of your diabetes management program. Having clear, accurate records allows you and your physician to make better decisions about your care.

Accurate blood sugar records will allow you and your physician to see early patterns or trends that will direct you to needed diet or medication changes.

Without adequate blood sugar records your physician will not be able to provide you with the advice you need to manage this disease. Showing up for a diabetes visit with your doctor without blood sugar records is like going to the mechanic to get your car repaired and not bringing the car—a waste of time for both of you.

The quality of your records is very important to the success of your doctor visit. Poor records are just about as bad as no records. Blood sugar records in your meter are not useful. Blood sugars on scraps of paper are rarely of any help. The perfect form has not been invented yet for recording on one page all the information needed to manage diabetes. But I do have some ideas that may help. The basic requirements include the date and blood glucose before meals, at bedtime, and at 3:00 AM. Then it would be helpful to superimpose diet and exercise information onto this form without making it too confusing (*see* Chapter 5 to learn about Xs for carbohydrates and Es for exercise).

When Do I Test? Before Meals? After Meals?

I have found the tests done before meals and at bedtime to be the most useful for adjusting insulin and oral medications. Getting the before-meal sugars into the target range of 90 to 130 mg/dl is a major challenge. If you are successful, your A1c will be at or very close to the target goal of 7. The after-meal test of <180 at one hour or <140 at two hours has helped me evaluate the effect of *portion size* or a type of food effect on a person's blood glucose. So if you want to know what that extra helping of mashed potatoes or that one small cookie does to your blood glucose, test at one or two hours and find out. This may be useful in helping you adjust your eating habits. Often it is not what you eat but how much of what you eat that causes the problem.

Portion size of carbohydrates is very often the main cause of erratic high blood glucose levels. Correcting the after-meal blood glucose may also become more important to your A1c results the closer you get to your target goal of 7.

In summary, the before-meal test will be the most useful to your doctor in helping you make necessary medication changes. The after-meal test will be most helpful to you for making adjustments in your eating habits.

Now here it is for the last time: before-meal and bedtime tests are most useful for adjusting medications; after-meal tests are useful in adjusting portion sizes and types of foods.

⇢3:00 AM blood glucose test? Why?

This is a time of day when we are most sensitive to glucose-lowering medications, especially sulfonylurea drugs (such as glipizide, glyburide, and glimepiride), and NPH insulin. In my experience, I have found that NPH insulin taken at dinnertime is not a good idea and is one common cause for 3:00 AM low blood glucose levels. This is related to its peaking effectiveness six to eight hours after being injected.

⇢How often should I test at 2:00 to 3:00 AM?

Test at least two different nights at about 3:00 AM if there are clues of low blood glucose levels such as:

- •Sweating in the middle of the night

- •Before-breakfast blood glucose tests below your target goal of 90

- •Erratic before-breakfast tests—on-target one day, high the next, etc.

Test one to two times a month if you take any sulfonylurea drug or if you take NPH insulin at dinnertime.

Sample blood sugar records are next.

Sample of Basic Form for Tracking Blood Sugar Records

Date	3:00 AM	Before Breakfast	Before Lunch	Before Dinner	Bedtime
2/28		93	112	135	110
2/29		99	121	157	143

Adding Diet and Exercise records
(*see* Chapter 5 for more information on Xs and Es)

Carbohydrates: number of servings __X__ Exercise __E__

Sample of Basic Form for Tracking Carbohydrate and Exercise Records

Date	AM		PM			
	1 2 3 4 5 6 7 8 9 10 11	12	1 2 3 4 5 6 7 8 9 10 11 12			
2/28	xxx		xxx E	x	xxxxx	x
2/29	xxx		xxx	xE xxxx		x

The goal is to have a form or forms that allow you and your physician to see blood sugar trends and patterns accurately.

Sample Combined Diet, Exercise, and Blood Sugar Record

Date	3:00 AM	Before Breakfast	Before Lunch	Before Dinner	Bedtime
2/28		93	112 E	135	110
		xxx	xxx x	xxxxx	x
2/29		99	121	157	143
		xxx	xxx	xE xxxx	x

David Calder, MD

Combined Diet, Exercise, and Blood Record

Date	3:00 AM AM	Before Breakfast	Before Lunch PM	Before Dinner	Bedtime
	1 2 3 4 5 6 7 8 9 10 11 12		1 2 3 4 5 6 7 8 9 10 11 12		

Chapter 5

Diet – My Thoughts on a Difficult Subject

What Are Those Xs and Es, Anyway?

Eating is a basic need that we all have; it is necessary for our survival. Eating is also associated with pleasure and good times with our friends and family. A person without diabetes can eat whatever is wanted, as much as is wanted, whenever it is wanted, and the Beta cells in his or her pancreas will produce just the right amount of insulin. This insulin will then allow conversion of the glucose that comes from carbohydrates in the meal to fuel for his or her body. The leftover glucose is stored as glycogen in the liver or added to existing fat deposits located in highly visible locations around the body, or, we could say, around his or her perimeter. Diabetes turns this normal system upside down.

Every person with diabetes mellitus has some degree of insulin deficiency. Some people will have a minor deficiency of insulin and others will have a severe lack of insulin that will require insulin replacement. A type 2 diabetes patient's problem is further complicated by having sluggish insulin release and by his or her body not responding correctly to the insulin that is produced. *A diabetes patient's body will no longer automatically adjust insulin production to carbohydrate intake. It is now necessary to adjust carbohydrate intake to match limited insulin production or insulin replacement. This becomes a major barrier that many diabetes patients will not overcome. The focus is now on using food—especially carbohydrates—and medications to control blood glucose levels.*

Thirty-five years of watching people with diabetes fail and succeed with food management has taught me a few things: the importance of portion size, portion size, portion size, portion size, (sorry, my fingers got stuck on----------PORTION SIZE----------), how to recognize foods that contain carbohydrates, and how eating habits, exercise, and blood glucose levels are interrelated.

The Importance of Portion Size

Most of us will not stay on a diet, and over time most of us will remain at about the same weight or slowly gain. We all seem to have pleasant little habits of a pinch of this and a bite of that associated with larger PORTION SIZES that we fail to recognize. Some of us do recognize the problem and fall off the wagon anyway. We frequently use excuses like stress, holidays, company, and vacations to get a little sloppy with our eating. Our problem with diets could be simple: it is more fun to eat than it is to be hungry. I think you can see from my discussion that I do not understand how to achieve long-term weight loss. One thing I do understand about diet and diabetes: erratic and uncontrolled portions of carbohydrate in our diet cause erratic and uncontrolled blood glucose levels.

You may have noticed that PORTION SIZE was only mentioned eight times in the above discussion. I was trying for ten. Here are the last two with a little flair.

Carbohydrate PORTION CONTROL IS IMPORTANT.

CARBOHYDRATE *portion control is important.*

How to Recognize Foods that Contain Carbohydrates

Most people do not understand which foods have carbohydrates. I bet you were thinking *pasta*. Pasta and sugar have been the most common answers when I ask patients to name four food groups that contain carbohydrate. A good friend of mine, Julie Scalisi, RD CDE, suggested an easy way to remember the answer: "If it grows out of the ground and we eat it, it has carbohydrate. Then just add milk."

Food groups that contain carbohydrates

- Grains

- Fruit

- Vegetables

- Milk

(Pay attention…there may be a pop quiz later.)

Carbohydrates and Your Blood Glucose Levels: How Eating Habits, Exercise, and Blood Glucose Levels are Interrelated

Many people are unaware of how much their current eating habits contribute to their high or unstable blood glucose levels. I believe that a good place to start is with carbohydrate recognition.

I have found that food diaries are difficult to keep; they are not tidy, and are often challenging to read. Food diaries also often obscure blood glucose readings. Making an X for each carbohydrate serving may work better. So how about putting an X on a piece of paper every time you eat a food that contains carbohydrate? Remember, this exercise is to just improve your carbohydrate recognition skills.

How you record this information is very important. Take a piece of notebook paper and put this information across the top:

DATE BREAKFAST LUNCH DINNER BEDTIME

I will now use myself as a typical example of diet ignorance. I was recently told that my fasting blood glucose level was slightly elevated to 115 mg/dl. This is not yet diabetes, but it is not normal. My options included starting Glucophage (metformin), increasing exercise, and reducing my weight.

I choose to increase exercise and lose weight. Here I am, a diabetes doctor in a very familiar situation. I know of good studies that demonstrate how weight loss and exercise can slow the progression to overt diabetes. I recognize that even though I eat a low-fat (almost vegetarian) diet, and I am very active (I'm a mass of solid muscle), I could stand to lose a few pounds.

So, what am I doing that may be contributing to this problem? It is time to take my own advice.

I will try to walk an extra thirty minutes each day, and I will take a closer look at my eating habits. My breakfast is usually granola cereal, a banana, and milk (that is only three Xs). My mid-morning snack is a protein bar; and lunch is usually a sandwich and milk (three more Xs). I have an apple or orange in the afternoon (another X) and vegetables at dinner (another X), plus a snack later (yet another X). I did this for a few days, and my diet record looked something like this:

Date	Breakfast		Lunch		Dinner	Bedtime
4/1	xxx	x	xxx	x	xx	x
4/2	xxx	x	xxx	x	xxx	x

This looks pretty good. I am very consistent. So what is the problem? Could it be...*portion size*? Oh no! Portion size.

Now things get a little tougher. I will need some additional tools. As I usually suggest to my patients, I will use measuring cups, and I will start reading food labels. A small scale may also be useful. I will download food lists for meal planning from www.lillydiabetes.com. Click "Diabetes Resources."

Now the first bad news about serving size: **one serving of carbohydrate is 15 grams** (that is one portion).

Now let us look at my carbohydrate intake after adding portion size to the equation. Since one X=one portion of carbohydrate or 15 grams, one half of an X=7.5 grams.

→**My breakfast:** I usually make coffee and eat a whole banana (30 grams of carbohydrate—whoops, that is two Xs); then I reach into the granola box and have two to three pinches of granola. To my surprise, each pinch was about a quarter of a cup or 15 grams of carbohydrate. (That is three more Xs, and I haven't even started breakfast yet.) Now that my pre-breakfast snack is over, I pour my usual man-sized bowl of granola. My typical portion turned out to be 2 cups—which equaled 120 grams of carbohydrate or eight normal servings. (Yipes! That is eight more Xs, and I haven't even added milk yet.) One cup of skim milk=12 grams of carbohydrate or about three quarters of an X. (Wow, I am glad that is over.) I repeated my usual breakfast evaluation for three days and found that I was fairly consistent. I was shocked to find that I was eating thirteen servings of carbohydrate (thirteen Xs) and did not even realize it.

→**My morning snack:** I usually have a high-protein bar (the label says 30 grams of carbohydrate or two more Xs) or a big apple (which is probably about 30 grams of carbohydrate also).

→My lunch: My favorite is a tuna sandwich and cup of skim milk. Each slice of bread is 15 grams of carbohydrate, according to the label. (I have found that some breads can be higher, so read labels carefully.) Skim milk is 12 grams. I am now up to nineteen servings of carbohydrates and the day is still young.

→My afternoon snack: I usually have a big orange or apple, about 30 grams of carbohydrate. I have just added two more Xs.

→My dinner: I often have a meatless burger patty; about 6 grams of carbohydrate; and 3 cups of stir fry vegetables, 9 grams of carbohydrate per cup. A cup of skim milk adds another 12 grams. This is a total of 45 grams=three servings or three more Xs. Wow. I am up to twenty-five servings of carbohydrate or twenty-five Xs, and it is now time for evening snack-o-rama. Five cups of popped popcorn (or five handfuls) adds another 24 grams of carbohydrate—at least another one and one half Xs. Another favorite is yogurt, 34 grams per cup. (I have found that the carbohydrate content of vegetables and yogurt can vary quite a lot depending on the ingredients. I suggest you pick your favorite foods and read the labels carefully.) By the end of a typical day, my total carbohydrate intake was about twenty-seven to twenty-eight servings of carbohydrates. I found that putting an X on my record sheet for each serving was easier and neater than keeping a food diary. It also helped me focus attention on carbohydrates and was easier for me to see variation in carbohydrate servings from day to day.

My food diary now looks something like this when I use portion size (15 grams per serving) to evaluate my carbohydrate intake:

Date	Breakfast	Lunch	Dinner	Bedtime
4/3	xxxxxxxxxxxx xx xxx	xx	xxx xx	x
4/4	xxxxxxxxxxx x xxx	xxx	xxxx	x

The other days are about the same until company looms—grandchildren and a horse show.

Date	Breakfast	Lunch	Dinner	Bedtime
5/5	xxxxxxxxxxxx	xx	xx xxxx	
5/6	xxxx	xxxx x	xxxxx	xx
5/7	xx xxx	xxxx xx	xxxx xxx	xxx

So much for my consistent day-to-day carbohydrate intake. If I had been on oral diabetes medication or insulin, what do you think would have happened to my blood glucose readings? I went back to my usual routine until...VACATION 5/27.

During my vacation I did not keep records, but "I watched my food." This is a familiar line that I have heard hundreds of times. I discovered that a large vanilla milkshake has 820 calories and 117 grams of carbohydrate. Wow. I did exactly what I have observed my patients doing for the past thirty-five years. There is more to this game than meets the eye. I gained three pounds on this little trip. There really is a big difference between knowing and doing, and it is now time for me to start doing. My life is on the line, and I alone am responsible for the outcome. (That was a little difficult to write, but I know that it is true. It is also true for you and your family and friends who have diabetes mellitus.)

At this point some people say, "This is too much trouble. So what if I lose a few years off my life? I probably won't be having much fun at that point in my life anyway." Diabetes does not usually work that way. It has been my observation that diabetes is like a vulture, picking away pieces of your body over many years until you are finally left with nothing. It is not a pleasant process and you don't get any "do over."

That's enough of this doom and gloom. Let's talk about the good news. You can beat this disease. The technology, medication, and knowledge are available. Your job is to understand the disease process and apply the medications and skills available to you. There will always be successes and failures in your efforts. Just do not quit. This is like hand-to-hand combat, and there is no second place. You might lose a few battles, but you can win the war. You must persist and never yield to this hateful disease. I have practiced diabetes medicine long enough to see a huge shift in my patients' problems. In the early years of my practice, many patients were sent to me for help in managing devastating complications of this disease. In the last fifteen-plus years, there has been a gradual shift to helping patients prevent such complications from ever developing. The prevention of complications is a lot more fun than treating complications.

Now let us get on with what I do best—telling other people what they need to do.

Quiz Time!

1. What are the three most important things to know about your diabetes food management? (If you do not know the answer to this question immediately, go back and read this section again.)

2. After you develop diabetes mellitus, it becomes necessary to adjust and

manage carbohydrate intake to match your limited insulin production or insulin replacement. True or False? (If you answered *false*, go back and read the first section again.)

Let's discuss why consistent day-to-day carbohydrate intake is so important. If you have type 1 diabetes, you will have—for the most part—no insulin production. If you have type 2 diabetes, you will have sluggish insulin release in response to an increase in blood glucose, limited insulin production, and probable tissue resistance to the limited insulin that you do produce. You may have noticed that limited insulin production is present in type 1 and type 2 diabetes mellitus. This fact is important when we talk about food, especially carbohydrate intake.

By now it is obvious that I have made or will make the same mistakes that you have already made or will make managing this difficult disease. It is therefore time to pick on Frank, a fictitious person who, much like the rest of us, is imperfect. We will have Frank switch from diet-controlled diabetes to oral diabetes medication and then finally to insulin.

The Exciting Story of Frank and Theola
Frank is a forty-five-year-old male. Weight 200 pounds. Height 5′ 9″.

BP 150/85
A1c 8
Cholesterol 210
Triglyceride 250
HDL 39
LDL 121
Creatinine 1.1

Frank has recently been started on lisinopril for his blood pressure, and simvastatin (Zocor) 40 mg for his cholesterol problem. He has been working with a dietitian and claims that he can recognize and measure portion sizes of carbohydrate. He has also read somewhere that he can just make an X for each carbohydrate serving on his record sheet rather that keeping a detailed list of foods. A sample of his record is below. He has been working on his diet for about a month.

Date	3:00 AM	Breakfast		Lunch		Dinner		Bedtime
5/1		121		164		142		151
		xxxxx	x	xxxx	x	xxxxx	x	x x
5/2		135		147		135		143
		xxxxx	x	xxxx	xE	xxxxx		xx

What is this E? It is a code letter we have not discussed yet, and it stands for thirty minutes of additional exercise. His blood glucose and food records are fairly stable until company comes, then diabetes management falls by the wayside.

Date	3:00 AM	Breakfast		Lunch	Dinner	Bedtime
5/3		133		191	202	196
		xxxxxx	xx	-	-	-
5/4		135			244	
		xx				
5/5		136				

Frank's company leaves and he almost gets back to his routine. He thinks, *No real damage done so why*

David Calder, MD

am I doing all of these blood tests and food diary stuff anyway? His wife, Theola, immediately reads his mind and screams, "Because the doctor said to!"

Frank takes his wife's advice and does a good job with records, much like those of 5/1 and 5/2. His doctor recommends that Frank start Glucophage on his next visit, starting with one pill each morning and adding one pill each week until he is taking two tablets in the morning and two tablets at dinner. If he has nausea, vomiting, or diarrhea at any dose level, he is to go back to the previous dose that did not cause symptoms, and stay at that dose for one week, then try to increase the dose again. If symptoms reoccur, he is to go back to the previous dose and stay there. He also is to inform his physician of the problem.

Frank has no problems with Glucophage and has an excellent response.

Date	3:00 AM	Breakfast	Lunch	Dinner	Bedtime
6/1		114	122	115	122

Frank switches to the Routine Monitoring Program.

Date	3:00 AM	Breakfast	Lunch	Dinner	Bedtime
6/3		112	118		
6/4		114		117	
6/5		110			115

Frank's A1c decreases to 6.8. All is well on the sugar front. (One little note about Glucophage: it is hard to get a low blood glucose with this medicine, but I have had patients have a mild hypoglycemia in the late afternoon after exercise.)

A few years go by and Frank is doing very well. His A1c has stayed at 7 or less, his BP is 125/80, and LDL cholesterol is 72. His triglyceride level is still a little high at 190, and his albumin/creatinine ratio is 22. Over all, a good job, but Frank has continued his routine glucose testing and has noticed a disturbing trend of increasing blood glucose levels, especially his before-breakfast results.

Date	3:00 AM	Breakfast	Lunch	Dinner	Bedtime
4/6		128	131		
4/7		136		115	
4/8		143			132
4/9		145	134		

Frank switches to the Diagnostic Program. *What is going on? I am not sick, I walk almost every day, and I am taking my Glucophage.*

Date	3:00 AM	Breakfast		Lunch		Dinner	Bedtime
4/10		145		141		135	157
		xxxx	x	xxxx	E	xxxxx	xx
4/11		144		155		123	152
		xxxx	x	xxxx	E	xxxxx	xxx

Frank makes an appointment and has an A1c done. It has increased to 7.9. His doctor explains that the disease has progressed and that his insulin deficiency is probably a little worse. He discusses adding another medication such as Actos (pioglitazone), Diabeta (Glyburide), Amaryl (glimepiride), Exenatide (Byeta), Sitagliptin (Januvia). Frank chooses Amaryl. His doctor explains that Frank is now at a little greater risk of low blood sugars than before, making consistent carbohydrate intake much more important. The Amaryl dose will be adjusted to correct his blood glucose to target range based on his current carbohydrate intake. If his carbohydrate level changes, his blood glucose will also change.

Let's see how Frank does after being started on 2 mg of Amaryl.

Date	3:00 AM	Breakfast		Lunch		Dinner	Bedtime
4/13		121		133		115	127
		xxxx	x	xxx	E	xxxxx	xx
4/14		111		122		119	128
		xxxx	x	xxxx	E	xxxxx	xx

Good result. Frank continues the Diagnostic Program for a few more days and then switches to the Routine Monitoring Program.

Date	3:00 AM	Breakfast	Lunch	Dinner	Bedtime
4/17		113	125		
4/18		107		118	
4/19		103			125

No problems. Everything is stable. A few months go by and a repeat: A1c is back down to 6.9. No problem with low blood glucose levels.

On 7/4 Company comes. Frank is up late talking and eating snacks.

Date	3:00 AM	Breakfast	Lunch	Dinner	Bedtime
7/5		153			
		x			

Frank decides to cut back on carbohydrates at breakfast because of the high sugar, and he takes a long walk with a friend. He then gets shaky, sweaty, and weak about 11:30 AM. His blood glucose is 65. He eats a candy bar and feels better. Then he has a big lunch of spaghetti and meatballs. Guess what? His blood glucose is 240 at dinnertime. What is going on?

Frank changed the deal. You may recall that he adjusted his Amaryl dose to match his carbohydrate intake. Frank changed his carbohydrate intake without any good way to change his medication because of its long effect time. It is impossible to adjust his oral medication to match the rapid changes made in his diet. I believe that trying to maintain carbohydrate intake at a consistent level is one of the most difficult parts of diabetes management. Is there a way around this problem? Yes, there is. Keep reading. Let's see how Frank does.

A few more years go by and again Frank's blood glucose levels increase and he again switches to his Diagnostic Program to evaluate the problem.

Date	3:00 AM	Breakfast	Lunch	Dinner	Bedtime
6/4		173	204	217	204
		xxxx x	xxxx	xxxxx	xx
4/11		219	248	197	215
		xxxx x	xxxx E	xxxxx	xx

This pattern continues with some of his before-breakfast glucose levels exceeding 240. His A1c is now 8.5. What do you think has happened? Frank's glucose levels are pretty consistent, which suggests that he is doing a good job with his diet. He is not ill. The most likely problem is worsening of his insulin production. He is still making insulin, just not enough. His doctor reviews Frank's options. He has already increased the Amaryl to 4 mg/day and further increase would probably not be of significant benefit. He discusses Byetta (exenatide), Januvia (sitagliptan) and Actos (pioglitazone) again but feels that Frank is too far along with his insulin deficiency to get the benefit he would need. The doctor suggests starting Lantus insulin, 10 units each morning, and adjusting the dose by a written schedule to correct his before-breakfast glucose to a target goal of 90 to 130. He explains that by correcting the breakfast sugar to target levels, Frank's diet and other medication might correct the other test.

Frank agrees and slowly increases his lantis insulin by protocol to 42 units which succeeds in correcting his before-breakfast blood glucose level into the target range. But the other before-meal results do not fall into place. His doctor explains that although Frank's outcome is not unusual, it was worth a try. His doctor then says, "I have some good news and some bad news. The good news is that we may be able to give you a lot of flexibility with your carbohydrate intake. You do an excellent job estimating your carbohydrate portions, so developing an insulin/carbohydrate ratio will be relatively easy."

Frank's response is, "What is that?"

The doctor replies, "The concept is pretty simple. You will take a fast-acting insulin before each meal or snack. We will start with 1 unit of insulin for every 15 grams (1 serving) of carbohydrate. This will give you a lot more freedom with your diet. For example, if you decide to eat 2 servings of carbohydrate for breakfast one day, you would take 2 units of fast-acting insulin. If you decide to eat 5 servings the next day, you would adjust the dose to 5 units. There will probably be some fine-tuning of the doses, but I think you will be happy with the results."

Frank listens carefully and says, "Thanks, but no thanks. Four and five shots each day? No way. I have a friend who takes 70/30 insulin at breakfast and dinner and just loves it. I would like to try 70/30 insulin."

His doctor says, "Fine! I will have my nurse teach you how use and adjust twice daily 70/30 insulin, and we will see how you like it. Good luck. By the way, you will really need to be consistent with your carbohydrate intake, especially your bedtime snack, as we help you adjust the dose. Be sure and check some 3:00 AM glucose levels to make sure they are staying above 90. You could replace your Lantus insulin tomorrow morning with 70/30 insulin. Also stop your Amaryl and we will just keep you on Glucophage and insulin."

A few months go by and everything is working well for Frank. He has had a few mild low blood glucose levels in the late afternoon but nothing to be concerned about. Then he wakes up one night sweating, shaking, and confused. His wife Theola has to help him get juice to correct his glucose level. Theola and Frank agree that having a low glucose at night was not one of their favorite evening activities.

Theola accompanies Frank to see his doctor next time. Her request is, "Tell us more about insulin/carbohydrate ratios and multiple insulin injections, and when we can start."

Frank mumbles under his breath, "That's easy for you to say…"

As usual, Frank does a good job with the multiple insulin injections and his A1c goes back down to 6.8.

Frank is now thinking about the pros and cons of an insulin pump. We will have to wait and see what happens.

So What is this E Thing?

Well, for most people it is thirty minutes of walking or jogging—over and above your usual daily routine. This is another thing that is difficult to do consistently. Having the big E on your glucose record may help serve as a reminder. From reviewing my own records, I have noticed that I am better at eating than I am at exercising. You may notice that trend also. What the heck—it gives us a little something to work on.

How About a Little Quiz?

1. Measuring and recording food amounts is difficult. True or False?

2. Often it is not what we eat but how much of what we eat that causes the problem. True or False?

3. Portion size and consistent carbohydrate intake are critical for controlling blood glucose levels. True or False?

4. Insulin/carbohydrate ratios are effective and give people with insulin-dependent diabetes more freedom with food choices and portion sizes. True or False?

5. Recording food diaries, carbohydrates in grams, blood glucose results, and exercise in a simple, understandable way is difficult. Using Xs and Es may be a better idea. True or False?

If you answered *true* to all the above, congratulations! If you missed one, go back and read the chapter again.

Chapter 6
Low Blood Sugars – No Fun Here

Hypoglycemia: Low Blood Sugar (a group of symptoms associated with a plasma glucose below 70 mg/dl)

L ow blood sugars are always a concern and need to be discussed with your physician. My personal contact with patients having hypoglycemia was not frequent. Mild episodes with shaking, anxiety, and sweating were usually treated by the patient and reported to me later during an office visit. Severe episodes with irritability, confusion, or even coma required immediate attention of a loved one, ambulance medic, or emergency or hospital nurse. My role in the immediate treatment was therefore minimal. I was usually called afterward to discuss the patient' medications and how to avoid another episode. Most of my patient contact was teaching someone how to adjust their insulin or oral medications to prevent low blood glucose levels from occurring. The type of hypoglycemia that I personally cared for was usually a hospitalized elderly person with recurrent prolonged hypoglycemia secondary to sulfonylurea medications such as glyburide and glimipiride (Amaryl). These patients often had mild impairment of their kidney function, and required intravenous glucose infusions for a few days.

→Common causes for hypoglycemia include:

1. Too much insulin or oral diabetes medications

2. Not eating enough food

3. Having had more exercise than usual

4. Alcohol on an empty stomach is not a good idea. This is very important and requires some discussion. When you are not eating, your liver is the primary source of glucose for your body. Alcohol is absorbed immediately from your stomach and turns off your liver's release of glucose into your blood stream. Guess what happens next? You are right if you said the blood glucose level also drops immediately and hypoglycemic symptoms start. This problem frequently occurs in the late afternoon, before dinner. The take-home message is: Don't drink alcohol on an empty stomach. Eat carbohydrate before having an alcoholic drink, and limit yourself to one drink only. Generally speaking, alcohol and diabetes is not a good combination.

→Basic presentations of low blood sugars:

• Plasma glucose below 70 mg/dl: mild symptoms of anxiety, sweating, shaking, palpitations, irritability, headache. As the glucose level gets lower, more severe symptoms develop, such as confusion and difficulty thinking, and can progress to coma.

Hypoglycemic Unawareness

A more severe form of hypoglycemia is *hypoglycemic unawareness*. With this situation the mild symptoms do not occur, and the person unknowingly slips into irritability, confusion, lack of awareness, difficulty thinking and speaking, stupor, and even coma. This is a severe problem and requires specific evaluation and rapid treatment. Hypoglycemic unawareness can result in automobile accidents and loss of driver's license. One of my patients suffered this form of hypoglycemia. She had her two children in her car and was found driving along a levee, totally unaware of where she was or what she was doing. This was a frightening experience for her and her family. Hypoglycemic unawareness requires frequent glucose monitoring and adjustment of insulin to completely avoid any low glucose readings. This will help regain some of the early warning symptoms of hypoglycemia. It is probably a good idea for anyone with insulin-dependent diabetes to test glucose level before driving.

Because of the risk of hypoglycemia, I have generally considered a home blood sugar test below 90 mg/dl as a reason to pay closer attention, start diagnostic blood sugar testing, and consider medication changes. Mild hypoglycemia symptoms or having a routine blood test below 70 mg/dl may be an early warning sign of a more severe low blood sugar to come.

Are there times of day when a person is at higher risk of low blood sugars? Yes.

- Late morning and late afternoon are higher risk and often associated with exercise.

 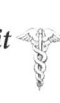

• 3:00 AM is a time of day when we are more sensitive to the effects of insulin.

There are a few clues to early-morning low sugars: unexplained sweating in the early-morning hours, before-breakfast blood sugars below 90, or wide swings in the before-breakfast blood sugars. In my experience, the use of NPH insulin or combinations that include NPH taken at dinnertime increases the risk. I also think it is a good idea to avoid short-acting insulins such as regular, and rapid acting insulins Humalog (insulin lispro), and NovoLog (insulin aspart) at bedtime unless you plan to check a 2:00 to 3:00 AM blood sugar.

If there is a concern, check a few 3:00 AM tests and discuss this problem with your physician.

Chapter 7
What Does That Test Mean?

This chapter discusses some of the tests that you will need to understand in order to successfully manage your diabetes. These tests include A1c, albumin/creatinine ratio, LDL cholesterol, HDL cholesterol, triglycerides, and total cholesterol. Have fun!

A1c (glycohemoglobin)

This test is an estimate of your average blood sugar tests over the previous two to three months, as well as being a marker of complication risk. This test reflects the amount of glucose that has attached itself to the hemoglobin in your red blood cells over last few months. Higher blood sugars = more attachment. The glucose attachment is permanent and stays with the red blood cell the remainder of its life span, which is about 120 days.

Now brace yourself for a more detailed explanation.

The A1c test gives an estimation of the average blood glucose during the eight to twelve weeks preceding the test. I have found from my own experience that pre-meal blood sugars of 90 to 130 will give an A1c result of about 7 and a lower risk of hypoglycemia. Always remember that your target goals for A1c have to balance the short-term risk of low blood sugars against the longer-term risk of high blood sugars. *Your physician's advice in this matter is essential.*

Achieving near normal A1c levels has been shown to reduce long-term complications of diabetes mellitus. Three major studies have demonstrated that good blood sugar control reduces complications. The Diabetes Control and Complication Trial (DCCT) in 1993[1] was done with type 1 diabetes patients and compared a control group with A1c levels of 9 to an intensively managed group with A1c levels of 7. The Kumamoto Study[2] with type 2 diabetes was reported a few years later and had similar treatment groups comparing patients with A1c levels of 9 to an intensive treatment group with A1c levels of 7. The United Kingdom Prospective Diabetes Study (UKPDS)[3] was reported in 1998. It, too, was done with type 2 diabetes patients and compared A1c levels 8 to 7. The results of the three are listed below.

	DCCT	Kumamoto	UKPDS
A1c reduced	9 to 7	9 to 7	8 to 7
Retinopathy reduced (eye damage)	63%	69%	17 to 21%
Nephropathy reduced (kidney damage)	54%	70%	24 to 33%
Neuropathy reduced (nerve damage)	60%		
Cardiovascular disease			16%

Demonstrating a decrease in the risk for cardio-vascular disease with improved A1c levels has been more difficult to prove. The 16% decrease in the UKPDS study was not statistically significant. However, in the same study when the results of intensive therapy with sulfonylurea/insulin were compared to metformin (Glucophage), there was a difference. Risk reduction compared to conventional treatment (A1c of 8 vs. A1c of 7).

Risk Reduction

	Sulfonylurea/in-sulin	Metformin
Microvascular (eye and kidney)	26%	29%
Myocardial in-farct	16%	39%
All cause mortal-ity	6%	36%

There is another interesting follow-up of patients with type 1 diabetes mellitus who were in the DCCT study. Over the seventeen years since the DCCT ended, the average A1c in the intensively managed group (A1c of 7) and the conventionally treated group (A1c of 9) had converged to about 8. There was a relative risk reduction of heart attacks, stroke, and cardiovascular death of 57% in the previously intensive control group. There has also been a ten-year follow-up of the UKPDS that was reported in the *New England Journal of Medicine*, September 10, 2008.[4] The between-group differences in A1c levels were lost after the first year. The benefits of intensive blood sugar control were not lost.

• The patients treated with sulfonylurea/insulin

▸Small vessel disease (eye and kidney damage) still reduced by 24%

▸Risk of myocardial infarction reduced by 15%

▸Death from any cause reduced by 13%

• UKPDS metformin (Glucophage) ten-year follow-up

▸Risk of myocardial infarction reduced by 33%

▸Death from any cause reduced by 27%

Two other studies, ACCORD (Action to Control Cardiovascular Risk in Diabetes) and ADVANCE (Action in Diabetes and Vascular Disease), will be completed within a few years of this book's publication. These studies may provide more insight into the effects of intensive blood sugar control on cardiovascular risk.

Albumin/Creatinine Ratio

This test is a marker of risk for kidney damage and heart disease. It indicates that there has been some degree of injury to your kidneys, causing them to leak protein into your urine. (*see* chart next page).

Now the good news: early, aggressive treatment can slow and even stop the progression of this problem. Control of blood sugars is very important. If possible, have an A1c goal of less than 7. Read the section on A1c in this chapter for more details. The use of medi-

Results	Name	Risk
0 to 30	Normal	
>30 to <300	microalbuminuria	10- to 200-fold risk of progressing to albuminuria
>300	albuminuria	A significant loss of kidney function may develop within the next 5 years

cations called ACE (angiotensin-converting enzyme) inhibitors is extremely important, as is the use of blood pressure (BP) control. Multiple medications to control BP are often needed. My next medication of choice is verapamil, a calcium channel blocker blood pressure medication that may enhance the ACE inhibitor effect of protecting our kidneys.

Having an albumin/creatinine ratio above 30 becomes another risk factor for heart disease. This is an indication to become more aggressive with control of blood sugar, blood pressure, and cholesterol.

My Thoughts on Lipids, Statins, and Diabetes

↪LDL, HDL, triglycerides

Almost all people with type 2 diabetes have an abnormal lipid profile and many people with type 1 diabetes have acceptable lipid results. It has been my observation that the changes in LDL cholesterol and triglycerides are often minimal and not aggressively treated. My opinion regarding lipid management has been influenced by four favorite studies and my own personal observations. The first study was reported by Haffner, et al., *New England Journal of Medicine*,

1998.[5] This study helped focus attention on the increased cardiovascular risk in people with type 2 diabetes. He compared non-diabetic subjects to subjects with type 2 diabetes and found a significant difference in cardiovascular events during a seven-year follow-up.

Incidence of cardiovascular (CV) events during a seven-year follow-up

	Non-diabetic subjects	Type 2 diabetes subjects
Myocardial infarction	3.5%	20.2%
Stroke	1.9%	10.3%
Death from all causes	2.1%	15.4%

I think most people will agree that there is increased cardiovascular risk associated with diabetes. The next question is, *How good are we at detecting heart disease in an asymptomatic patient with type 2 diabetes?* Unfortunately, we do not do well in this area. The DIAD Study (Detection of Ischemia in Asymptomatic Diabetes) reported their findings in *Diabetes Care*, 2004.[6] This study found that 22% of these asymptomatic patients with type 2 diabetes had silent myocardial ischemia. They concluded that one in five asymptomatic patients with type 2 diabetes could have silent myocardial ischemia.

Is there something we can do about this? Yes.

⇥The inside story about LDL cholesterol

What if I told you about an inexpensive, safe medication that can significantly reduce the risk of developing cardiovascular disease? Would you take it?

These medications do exist. These antihyperlipidemic agents (HMG-CoA reductase inhibitors) are called *statins*. There are many drugs in this family. Some of the more common ones are: Zocor (simvastatin), Lipitor (atorvastatin), Mevacor (lovastatin), Pravachol (pravastatin), and Crestor (rosuvastatin).

I have two favorite studies that point out just how effective these medications are in preventing cardiovascular disease. The first one is The Heart Protection Study.[7] This study demonstrated substantial benefit to patients with diabetes, It also demonstrated benefit to patients regardless of age or sex. Their conclusion was that taking 40 mg of simvastatin daily would reduce LDL cholesterol by 38.8 mg/dl and reduce the rates of heart attacks, strokes, and revascularizations by about one-quarter. Another way of looking at their data is to say, that five years of simvastatin use would prevent about 54 people per 1000 from suffering a major vascular event. This study also demonstrates that there is probably not a threshold below which lowering LDL would not reduce risk. In this study, lowering LDL from below 116 mg/dl to below 77 mg/dl reduced vascular risk by one-quarter, which is similar to the proportional reduction in risk produced by a 39 mg/dl reduction at higher LDL cholesterol concentrations.

Another study, called The CARDS study (Collaborative Atorvastatin Diabetes Study Primary—prevention of cardiovascular disease with atorvastatin in type 2 diabetes)[8] had equally impressive results. This study included 2838 patients 40 to 75 years old with no documented previous history of cardiovascular disease, an LDL cholesterol of below 161 mg/dl, triglyceride below 597 mg/dl, and one of the following: retinopathy, albumin urea, hypertension, or current smoking. The treatment group received atorvastatin 10 mg/day and experienced significant benefit.

Summary of CARDS study benefits

- Acute coronary heart disease events reduced by 36%

- Coronary revascularizations reduced by 31%

- Rate of stroke reduced by 48%

- Death rate reduced by 27%

Over all, treatment would be expected to prevent at least 37 major vascular events per 1000 people treated for 4 years with atorvastatin 10 mg/day. There are several other studies demonstrating the value of statins. I have included some of them in the References provided in the back of this book: ASCOT study,[9] PROVE-IT study,[10] ARBITER study,[11] REVERSAL study.[12]

My favorite line from The CARDS study is, "The debate about whether all patients with type 2 diabetes warrant statin treatment should now focus on whether any patient can reliably be identified as sufficiently low risk for this safe, efficacious treatment to be withheld."

Unfortunately, many patients with diabetes are not treated with statins. I became more aware of this a few years ago when John Nelson, PA, and I noticed that many patients with diabetes who were admitted to our hospital for coronary bypass surgery were not taking any cholesterol-lowering medication. We took a closer look (with John doing all the work) and found that only 37% of diabetes patients admitted for a coronary bypass were on a statin. These results were similar to a study reported in the *New England Journal of Medicine*, volume 350.[10] They found that only 25% of patients admitted with acute coronary syndrome were on a statin.

I am sure there are many reasons for the under-treatment of lipid disorders in people with diabetes. However, and regardless of the cause, I think this under-treatment could be corrected by having physicians and their patients establish specific targets for all their diabetes laboratory test results. If they agree on goals, then it is just a matter of both parties doing what is necessary to reach the goals. I personally feel that a target LDL of 70 mg/dl or less is the level of optimal benefit. For more details, please refer to Chapter 2: Setting Goals and Talking to Your Doctor.

➤**Does size really matter?**
There is one last interesting thing about LDL cholesterol. Size does matter. LDL particles come in various sizes from small and dense to larger, less dense particles. The smaller LDL size is associated with a higher risk of vascular disease. One thing that promotes the conversion of the large LDL to the bad small LDL is elevation of triglyceride levels. The change to small LDL starts at triglyceride levels of about 100 mg/dl. This effect appears to be reversible. Reducing triglycerides to the target goal of 150 is effective in increasing conversion from the smaller LDL back to the larger, safer size. Bigger LDL is better. Don't overlook elevated triglyceride levels.

Chapter 8
The Definition of "Long-term" from an Old Geezer's Perspective

I have spent most of my years helping people with diabetes avoid the "long-term" complications of this disease. I really hadn't thought about the actual meaning of those words until recently, but I have noticed that "long-term" has gotten shorter as I have matured.

One morning I was sitting in my office in deep thought about the real meaning of *long-term* and how it might affect diabetes treatment decisions. I was trying to determine where I could actually see and talk to "old people." Visiting a nursing home seemed like a good idea. Then I heard a noise in my family room. I went into stealth mode and peaked around the corner and to my surprise, there was one (an old person) sitting on my couch and watching my TV. I slipped on my trifocals, slapped in my hearing aids, turned up the volume, and went in to investigate.

I quickly discovered that the old person sitting there was my wife. I wondered for a moment how old age could have happened to her and totally missed me. (As you might expect, I did not mention that last thought.) I then explained to her what I was thinking about, and she politely responded, "You dummy, everyone you know is old. Just pick up the phone and call a few of our remaining relatives." I took her advice, remembering a plaque she has hanging on the wall that says, "If at first you don't succeed, try it your wife's way." My wife said that to her, *long-term* meant about ten years.

I called my older brother, and he and his wife Evelyn (lovingly know as "Jake & them") agreed that there is no *long-term*. I then asked him about his greatest fear, and I got the expected older-brother response, "I have no fear." He later changed that and admitted that he had one fear—kidney stones.

My family interviews continued. My brother-in-law, Tom, quickly answered, "Two days." My wife's cousin, Leona, said, "About five years," also pointing out that nothing tasted good anymore. Last was a forty-something cousin who said, "about forty years." With these highly unscientific results in mind, I decided to look at some of my favorite studies from a different point of view. How long does someone have to follow the recommended program before seeing results? Continuing along this same unusual path, I decided that since this was my idea, I would do it my way, so I only selected studies that I liked and that agreed with my opinion. I included two other criteria. The study had to have a graph that looked something like this and was easily found in my files.

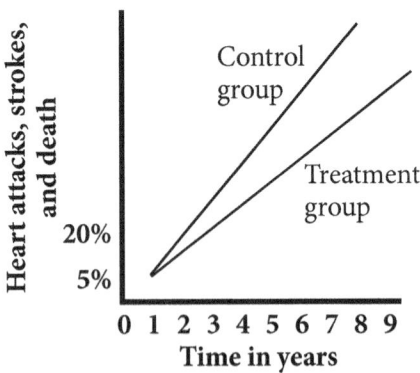

⇸Study results: use of statins to treat LDL cholesterol and reduce cardiovascular disease risk

- Heart Protection Study. *Lancet* 361.[7] Simvastatin 40 mg vs. placebo. At about one and one-half years, the simvastatin group started showing decreased vascular events.

- CARDS study. *Lancet* 364.[8] Atorvastatin 10 mg vs. placebo. In less than one year, there was a beginning reduction in major cardiovascular events. There are also studies with high dose atorvastatin (Lipitor) showing benefit within days of starting the medication.

⇸Study results: use of ACE inhibitors

- HOPE study (Heart Outcomes Prevention Evaluation) *NEJM* 342.[13] Ramipril 10 mg vs. placebo. Primary outcome myocardial infarction/stroke/cardiovascular death. There was a 15% event reduction in one year.

- REIN study (Ramipril Efficacy in Nephropathy) *Lancet* 354.[14] Ramipril 10 mg vs. placebo. Ramipril reduced the progression to proteinuria by 58%. The benefits started showing up in less than one year.

⇸Study results: blood glucose control

- UKPDS study group. *Lancet* 352.[15] A1c of 7 vs. A1c of 8. Reduction in microvascular disease (eye, nerve, and kidney damage) started improving at about two and one-half years.

➤Study results: blood pressure control

- UKPDS study group *BMJ* 317.[16] Also the above Lancet report. Mean BP 144/82 vs. 154/87. The lower BP group had a 24% reduction for any diabetes-related outcome, 34% reduction in death related to diabetes, 37% reduction in microvascular disease, 44% reduction in strokes, and 56% reduction in heart failure. I could not find a timeline to show length of time to an expected benefit, but the results here prove the importance of controlling blood pressure.

There is a motive to this madness. The prevention of long-term diabetes-related complications does not have to be that long-term. Some risk reduction starts very soon after beginning a medication. This means to me that age alone is not a reason for denying treatment to someone.

Diabetes in an Aging Loved One

Diabetes in an aging loved one may present difficult problems for families. I have observed that providing care frequently falls to a daughter. I can still picture these exhausted, frightened daughters, concerned that they were unable to do more for their mother or father. Those were difficult times for all concerned, including me. I found that I was better at attacking a problem than regrouping and changing tactics. I soon realized that aging has a way of affecting us all. According to my brother Jake (formally known as John Calder, DDS), "Aging is the great equalizer." Aging also teaches us to make decisions based on how things *are* rather than how we want things to be.

Getting older is sometimes associated with the loss of ability to consistently manage medication or maintain a consistent food intake. Such problems are exaggerated if the person has diabetes mellitus. Many of the diabetes-associated problems revolve around food. Friends and family may not understand the impact that erratic food intake has on blood glucose levels. They may not understand how the special treat bought or made out of love for that person is contributing to higher, often erratic glucose levels. The situation is often made worse by a family or loved one's expectations versus the reality of what can be accomplished under the circumstances. It has also been my experience that the older person who is in this situation is often asymptomatic and not too concerned that a problem even exists. The caregiver, usually a family member, is the person concerned about uncontrolled blood sugars. A common call to me, especially on weekends, was from a family member or nurse wanting something done for high sugars.

To me this is where the definition of long-term and the consequences of high blood sugars come into play and join the rules of reality. The immediate effect of high blood sugars becomes more important and the long-term risk of high blood sugars become less important. Some of the immediate effects of high blood glucose include blurred vision, increased frequency of urination, increased thirst, dehydration, tiredness, and perhaps decreased mental acuity. Some of these problems are more difficult to detect than others. Low blood glucose levels also now become more of an issue. We, as health care providers, often have to reassess patients' abilities to care for themselves and reset the management goals to avoid the acute symptomatic effects of high and low blood glucose levels.

The next step is to focus attention on the caregivers and other family members. Help them maximize the use of in-home care, assisted living situations, or nursing home care if needed to give them a little relief from this stressful situation. Explain the new management goals to the patient's family and discuss how they can be involved to help meet the new goals. This does not mean we should abandon all efforts to attain the best blood glucose control possible under the circumstances. For example, Lantus insulin is often a good choice to safely improve the before-breakfast blood glucose levels. Lantus insulin can be given one time daily in the morning along with oral diabetes medications without too much additional strain for the care provider.

Well, that is enough of this down-in-the-mouth talk. Let me tell you a story about another side of getting old. A number of years ago our hospital required doctors in the internal medicine department to review a certain number of hospital charts for various problems and to make a report to the department. We were divided into groups of three or four doctors and asked to choose a topic. One group decided to review surgery in the aged. They first had to set criteria for the term *aged*. As I recall, they decided 92 years old and above was appropriate. They were sure that they had outdone the system. They were sure there would be few if any charts to review, thus a small time commitment and a brief report to the group were all that would be required.

The day for chart review came and they were shocked at what they saw. Stacks and stacks of charts to review. It took a little while to overcome their initial surprise, and then they discovered a new dimension to getting old. There are a lot of healthy old people out there. They discovered that many were independent and having a good time. They also found that most of them survived major surgery and returned to their own homes. This provided some necessary insight for everyone in the department. *Getting old does not always mean poor health.*

Chapter 9

"Long-term" Risk Factor Management – Tracking Diabetes-related Data

Who is Responsible for What?
Like you, I have been given a beautiful, complex, finely tuned body that requires periodic repair and maintenance. Also like you, I am pretty good about keeping up on the exterior care— taking a bath, brushing my teeth, and combing all four of my remaining hairs. For some people, however, interior care is often felt to be the responsibility of someone else, such as a doctor or other health care professional. Just as you cannot expect your doctor to help you with bathing and brushing your teeth every day, you cannot expect your doctor to assume complete responsibility for your body's interior maintenance.

I believe that we doctors are good at making a diagnosis, solving a problem, and making treatment recommendations—if the problem is put in front of us by someone else. If you have diabetes, that someone else is you. You cannot afford to take the Greyhound approach and "Sit back, relax, and leave the driving to us." This is a time when you have slip into the driver's seat. I do, as you might expect, have some studies and clinical observations to back up this opinion.

I recently reviewed an article published in the *Journal of the American Medical Association* (*JAMA*).[17]

This article pointed out that only 7.3% of people with diabetes were meeting the standards of care recommended by the American Diabetes Association for A1c, LDL cholesterol, and blood pressure. That means that 92.7% were *not* meeting recommended goals. Another study, published in *Practical Diabetes International*,[18] found that only 16.2% of patients with type 2 diabetes mellitus actually carried out recommendations given to them by their health care provider, and health care providers felt that only 3% of patients followed their directions. I have made some personal clinical observations that confirmed my opinion that we as patients and physicians do not get the job done as well as we could.

I noticed that many of the diabetes patients admitted to our hospital for coronary bypass surgery were not on any lipid-lowering medication. A few years ago John Nelson, PA, and I looked more closely at 121 of these patients and found that only 37% were taking any cholesterol-lowering medication. My medical group started a diabetes management program and enrolled over 3000 patients. I noticed that 70% of these patients had a lipid profile done that year, with 70% having an LDL cholesterol of over 100 mg/dl, but only 42% were on a statin (cholesterol-lowering medication). A study reported in the *New England Journal of Medicine* (*NEJM*)[10] found only 25% of patients with diabetes admitted with acute coronary syndrome were on statins.

I also noticed that tests (A1c, lipid profiles, and albumin/creatinine ratio) that were automated with computerized reminders sent out to patients actually got done about 68% of the time. Other jobs that were more dependent on the patient and physician to complete were done less often. Only 40%

of eye and foot exams were completed; LDL <100 was 39%; A1c <7 only 38% of the time; albumin/creatinine ratio >30 being treated with an ACE inhibitor or ARB (Angiotensin II receptor blocker) was 46%; and BP <130/80 was completed less than 24% of the time. I think it is clear that there is room for improvement. How can we as patient and doctor do a better job? As you may expect, I do have another opinion. I believe it is due to a failure to establish who is responsible for what. Just as doctors cannot take care of your exterior body maintenance, we also cannot assume full responsibility for your interior maintenance.

The diabetes doctor's office visit is a complex interaction of patient expectations of what a doctor can do and the reality of what can be delivered. Often there is confusion about who actually manages this disease. If the patient's expectation is to turn this illness over to his or her doctor, or if the doctor thinks he or she can actually manage this disease for the patient, they will both be disappointed. Day-to-day diabetes management is extremely difficult to do over a long period. It is not just taking a pill or a shot and then getting well. Diabetes is a day-in/day-out job of controlling food intake, exercise, and medication. This is all done by the person with diabetes and not by their physician. I have listed below my suggestions for the "who is responsible for what" idea.

It is Your Life: Take Charge
→ **The physician's role is that of an advisor who provides three things:**

> 1. Expert advice and/or access to someone who can provide expert advice about the disease and medications.

Diabetes physicians should take the time to review and discuss laboratory tests and home glucose test results. Patients work hard on their home test records, and they are proud of their accomplishments or want help understanding the results. I am sorry to say that physicians often just take a quick look at the results, set them aside, and go on with their agenda. This is a huge mistake. This action is equivalent to taking a quick glance at a hand-drawn picture your child proudly hands to you, giving it a *hmmm*, and then tossing it in the trash. The message to the patient is that testing is of no value, so why do it. Patients need to understand that their home testing efforts are an important part of their care. Doctors know this, but failure to pay attention to home testing records was one of the most common complaints patients made to me about their *previous* physician.

2. Access to diabetes-management education and necessary laboratory tests

3. Establishing treatment goals with patient and providing a structure for long-term tracking and follow-up of important management tests and procedures

↛ **The patient's responsibilities include:**

1. Being informed about diabetes. Go to diabetes education classes!

2. Having a clear understanding of the role carbohydrate intake plays in blood glucose control, especially portion size and consistent day-to-day carbohydrate intake (*see* Chapter 5)

3. Doing daily exercise

4. Doing appropriate home glucose testing and keeping accurate, readable records (*see* Chapters 3 and 4)

5. Setting diabetes-management goals with your physician (*see* Chapter 2)

6. Tracking long-term data of important management tests and procedures to ensure that every test is done on a consistent basis (*see* Chapter 9)

7. Asking your physician about a diabetes specialist in your area. (Do not hesitate to request a referral if you feel it is necessary. Remember, your physician has your best interest in mind and will generally be happy to get any advice that will help you do a better job of managing your diabetes.)

You may have noticed that setting goals, getting appropriate tests done, and tracking data are shared responsibilities. Physicians and medical groups often try to assume full responsibility for getting tests done and tracking the results. It bears repeating that this effort will not be 100% effective without 100% patient participation. We as physicians can set up exams and order tests, but without our patients' buy-in to the process, the procedures will not get done. Remember that diabetes is not a spectator sport. Diabetes management requires your full participation. I don't think anyone really wants this diabetes-management job, but if it has fallen into your life, don't despair; instead, realize that you have been given an opportunity to discover your real strengths to persist and defeat a hateful, unforgiving opponent.

It is now your privilege to take on another job—tracking your long-term laboratory and procedure results. This is another difficult but essential job that will help you and your doctor know when to schedule needed tests. You will also be able to see at a glance how you are doing at meeting your long-term management goals. I have included a form that you may find useful. Please make copies and improvements.

Risk Factor Management Form					
Suggested form for tracking long-term factors					
Date					
BP					
A1c					
Alb/ creat. ratio					
Choles- terol					
LDL chol.					
HDL chol.					
Triglyc- eride					
Aspi- rin use yes/no					
Weight					
Waist size					
Foot exam (each year)					
Eye exam (each year)					

Chapter 10

The Office Visit (Putting it All Together), Plus a Surprise Visit with Mrs. Do-Right

I have thought about diabetes mellitus from the perspective of **"who is responsible for what,"** and I believe most of the responsibility for a successful office visit falls on the patient's shoulders. We physicians are very good at dealing with specific issues placed in front of us. Your job as a patient is to recognize when there is a problem and to then bring it up with your physician. This is not as hard as it sounds. It all starts with setting management goals and targets (*see* Chapter 2). I've talked about goals and targets all through these chapters, but I'll say it again here because it is the major point of this book: **if you and your doctor have agreed on goals, then any result that does not meet those goals is a problem that has to be discussed and resolved.**

I can tell you which results will be the most difficult to correct and may require some compromise. Raising HDL and lowering triglycerides to the target range will be difficult—at times impossible. Getting blood pressure to target can be a real challenge and often requires two or three different medications. For some reason, starting ACE inhibitors for confirmed albumin/creatinine ratios over 30 will sometimes be overlooked. The other big one is having type 2 diabetes and not being on a statin drug. I believe that every person with type 2 diabetes and some people with type 1 diabetes could benefit from taking a statin, a cholesterol-lowering medication (*see* Chapter 7).

Again, tracking tests and procedures (see Chapter 9) is your privilege. Of singular importance is the diabetes foot exam—probably one of the most overlooked procedures in diabetes care. You can fix that problem by scheduling this exam once a year. I have tried many approaches to this problem and one of the most frustrating was putting a sign in every exam room, asking each patient to remove their shoes. A common occurrence for me was that after having just spent thirty-five minutes discussing a diabetes problem with a patient, it would be 5:55 PM and I'd be heading for the door when the patient would point at his or her feet and say, "Why did you have me remove my shoes? Aren't you going to check my feet?" (It did not take long for me to remove those pesky signs.)

It is a good idea to check your feet regularly. If you have loss of sensation or poor circulation in your feet, have your doctor look at your feet more often. Just tell the doctor up front that you would like to have a quick look at your feet. A full diabetes foot exam needs to be an annual, scheduled visit. This exam is a little more complex and takes more time. This test involves checking for sensation loss, which includes the use of a 5.07 monofilament, close evaluation of the skin, and a check for pulses. Sometimes finding pulses in feet, especially women's feet, takes a little time. I am not sure why; it could be as simple as women just having smaller arteries.

The final test that you are 100% responsible for is getting your annual diabetes eye exam done by an ophthalmologist. Don't forget to share the results with your doctor at your next diabetes office visit.

I think you can appreciate the large number of details and the complexity of a "simple" diabetes office visit. I have experienced many office and hospital diabetes visits over the last forty years. Some visits were better than others.

Unproductive visits were similar in many regards. Patients' concerns were usually about a high A1c result and/or high or erratic blood sugar test. Home plasma glucose test results were either inadequate or absent, food and exercise records almost never present. I would then have to rely on their recall of glucose test results and diet habits. This information was generally vague and not helpful. The only accurate data was an A1c test done at the time of their visit. This test would just confirm that their diabetes was not well controlled. Without accurate data, I would have difficulty making any useful management suggestions. Often we would discuss the value of home testing records, and I would refer them to one of our diabetes educators for more training. I found that many patients wanted to do a good job but had not received adequate diabetes self-management instructions. Other people had been trained but chose not to participate fully in home diabetes management. Overall, this was an unsatisfactory visit for the patient and me. Unfortunately, this type of visit occurs in doctors' offices every day.

Contrast this mediocre visit with that of a patient who is a full partner in his or her own care. Such a patient presents differently, making sure to have a current A1c test result as well as home glucose and diet records. This patient's questions are different. He or she may say, "Doctor, my recent A1c test result was 8, and I have noticed that my before-meal tests have been above my target goals. Here are my diet and home glucose test results. Can you help me fix this problem?"

What do you think the doctor's response will be? I can tell you. First the doctor will faint, and then, after getting up off the floor, he or she will do everything possible to help that patient solve the problem.

I have listed a few suggestions below that may help you prepare for a visit related to high home glucose test results. Please review Chapter 2 for more information.

Scheduling the Diabetes Office Appointment

- Be very clear about the reason for your visit. For example, "My before-breakfast and before-lunch home glucose tests are above my target goals."

- Schedule a thirty-minute visit, if possible.

- Request a current A1c before the office visit, if needed. It should be available at the time of your visit.

Preparing for the Visit

- Have your home glucose test results with you. Please review chapter 3 for more information, if needed.

- Have diet and exercise records available. Please see Chapters 4 and 5 for more information, if needed.

The Visit

Focus on the reason for the visit—diabetes management problems. Do not bring up distracting issues such as tiredness or a nagging backache. If you have additional problems, other than an emergency, schedule a separate visit to discuss those problems. Be sure to schedule another visit to follow up on recommendations made for today's diabetes management problem.

Office visits often include blood pressure discussion, and BP results are available at the end of each visit. Also at the end of the visit, you may ask about scheduling your yearly foot and eye examinations, if they have not been done yet.

I recommend keeping track of your own risk factors and lab results by using the Risk Factor Management Form (at the end of Chapter 9), and scheduling visits to discuss results that are not at target goals.

And now for a little visit with Mrs. Do-Right…

•••

Putting It All Together With Mrs. Do-Right

Mrs. Do-Right is a thirty-eight-year-old female, height 5' 2", 160 pounds, DM (diabetes mellitus) × eight years, BP 150/95 with home BP test about the same. Her medication is Glucophage 1000 mg twice daily, Amaryl 4 mg/day, lisinopril 10/day, and Zocor 20 mg/day.

↬Dr. Calder and Mrs. Do-Right

Dr. Calder: I have reviewed your medication list. How can I help you?

Mrs. Do-Right: My A1c was 8 last month. I would like to get it back down to 7. My blood tests have been increasing over the last few months.

Dr. Calder: Do you have your home test results?

Mrs. Do-Right: Yes, here are my most recent tests. They are all a little higher than my target goal of 90 to 130 before meals. I have noticed a slight decrease on my exercise days. I have marked them with an E. I have also started marking my carbohydrate servings with an X. (She hands the records to the doctor).

Dr. Calder: WOW, great records!

(Doctor faints).

Nurse Nice pops through the exam-room door with a cool, damp cloth and places it carefully on the doctor's brow and says, "This seems to be happening more frequently since everybody started reading some new book called *The Diabetes Office Visit.*"

(Doctor gets up, revived by the cool, swift actions of Nurse Nice.)

Dr. Calder: WOW! Very good data. Your glucose levels are stable, suggesting that your carbohydrate intake is consistent. Your insulin production may have decreased a little more. What type of diet do you follow?

Mrs. Do-Right: Low fat. And I try to increase foods with Omega 3 fatty acids. I try to keep my carbohydrate servings fairly constant with each meal. I have three servings of carbohydrate at breakfast and three to four with lunch and dinner.

Dr. Calder: Do you pay attention to portion size?

Mrs. Do-Right: No. Do you have any suggestions that will help me reach blood sugar goals?

Dr. Calder: Yes. I would start working on portion size. Would you like to talk to a dietitian?

Mrs. Do-Right: I think I will work on this myself first. I have measuring cups and a Lilly diet sheet, and I will pay closer attention to food labels.

Dr. Calder: I suggest we add another medication. I think Byetta would be a good choice. Byetta (exenatide) is excellent medication. It is the first incretin mimetic therapy that has become available. It works similarly to GLP-1 (glucagon-like peptide-1), a normal hormone produced in the intestinal track. It has some very desirable effects, including improved insulin production and glucose-sensitive insulin release. It helps restore the first-phase insulin release that is impaired in type 2 diabetes. Byetta reduces glucagon, which is abnormally elevated in type 2 diabetes and causes increased release of glucose from the liver. In addition, it slows emptying of the stomach and helps reduce food intake. Weight loss is another good benefit of this medication. Byetta has to be injected twice daily and can have a side effect of nausea. We usually start with the smallest dose. In general, I have found that it is very well tolerated. There is another newer injectable, Victoza (liraglutide), that is similar to Byetta and can be given just one time daily.

Mrs. Do-Right: That sounds good. Are there other options?

Dr. Calder: Yes there are a number of options. Actos (pioglitazone) is another good choice. It works by improving the efficiency of how the cells in your body handle glucose. Sometimes there can be a little weight gain and/or slight edema with this drug. There are a number of new medications, such as Januvia (sitagliptin) and Onglyza (saxagliptin). Both of these oral medications have the same effects as Byetta—they just work by a different mechanism. I have not used this medication yet but I think it has excellent potential. It has the some of the same effects as Byetta. It works by a different mechanism interfering with an enzyme that breaks down GLP-1 in the body. This will prolong the effect of your normal GLP-1. As I mentioned, other than weight loss it has effects similar to those of Byetta. I understand that it is less effective with weight loss. We could increase Amaryl, but there is very little benefit in going to 8 mg/day. Lantus insulin is a good choice and will always work, and we could go to this if Byetta fails.

Mrs. Do-Right: I will go with Byetta.

Dr. Calder: Good. My nurse will teach you how to use it. Reduce your Amaryl by half and continue to reduce by half if you have any blood sugar below 90. Our goal is to get rid of Amaryl, if possible.

(They discuss side effects.)

Dr. Calder: Also, your BP is elevated—could you increase Lisinopril to 20 mg/day and have a return visit in two weeks?

Mrs. Do-Right: Yes. Also, on our next visit, I would like to discuss my cholesterol management and other long-term management goals. Here is a copy of my long-term goals. My diabetes foot exam will also be due soon.

Dr. Calder: Be sure and schedule a thirty minute visit next time, and we will try to get everything done then.

Dr. Calder smiles, jumps in the air, clicks his heels together, and says, "Nurse Nice, bring on the next patient. I think this stuff actually works!"

This book and its last chapter are a reflection of experiences and ideas that came from working with many wonderful people who happened to have diabetes. I learned so much about life and diabetes from my patients. I learned to appreciate the inner toughness and strengths of the frailest person. I learned how these attributes would always rise to the surface when circumstance demanded their presence.

I hope that after you read this book, you will appreciate the difficulties and complexities of diabetes care. This book includes my observations and more than a few opinions that you are free to accept or reject. The main purpose is to improve diabetes care conversation with your doctor and for you to become a better participant in your own care. I hope this book helps you understand that you can win the battle with this disease. Just be smart, accept responsibility, persist and never yield to this hateful disease. Be a full partner in your diabetes care. Your health is too important to trust to someone else.

Good luck!

—Doctor Calder

Appendix I
Notes and References

Notes

1. Diabetes Control and Complication Trial Group. "The Effect of Intensive Treatment of Diabetes on the Development and Progression of Long-Term Complications in Insulin-Dependent Diabetes Mellitus." *New England Journal of Medicine* 329 (September 30, 1993): 977–986. [DCCT]

2. Ohkubo Y., et al., "Intensive insulin therapy prevents the progression of diabetic microvascular complications in Japanese patients with non-insulin-dependent diabetes mellitus: a randomized prospective 6-year study." *Diabetes Research and Clinical Practice* 28 (May 1995): 103–117.

3. UK Prospective Diabetes Study (UKPDS) Group 33. "Intensive blood-glucose control with sulphonylureas or insulin compared with conventional treatment and risk of complications in patients with type 2 diabetes." *Lancet* 352 (September 12, 1998): 837–853.

4: *New England Journal of Medicine*, September 10, 2008 [follow-up of UKPDS study]

5: Haffner, SM., et al. "Mortality from coronary heart disease in subjects with type 2 diabetes and in non-diabetic subjects with and without prior myocardial infarction." *New England Journal of Medicine* 339 (1998): 229–234. [Haffner study]

6.The DIAD Study. "Detection of Silent Myocardial Ischemia in Asymptomatic Diabetic Subjects." *Diabetes Care* 27, no. 8 (August 8, 2004): 1954–1961. [DIAD Study]

7. Heart Protection Study Collaborative Group. "MRC/BHF Heart Protection Study of cholesterol-lowering with simvastatin in 5963 people with diabetes: a randomised placebo-controlled trial." *Lancet* 361 (June 14, 2003): 2005–2016. [Heart Protection Study]

8. *Lancet* 364 (August 21, 2004): 685–696. [CARDS Study]

9. *Lancet* 361 (2003); 1149–1158. [ASCOT Study]

10. *New England Journal of Medicine* 350, no. 15 (April 8, 2004): 1495–1504. [PROVE IT Study]

11. *Circulation* 106 (2002): 2055–2060. [ARBITER Study]

12. *Journal of the American Medical Association* 251 (2004): 1071–1080. [REVERSAL Study]

13. HOPE study (Heart Outcomes Prevention Evaluation) *New England Journal of Medicine* 342 (2000): 145–153

14. REIN study (Ramipril Efficacy in Nephropathy) *Lancet* 354 (1999): 359–364

15. UKPDS study group. *Lancet* 352 (1998): 837–853

16. UKPDS study group *British Medical Journal* 317 (1998): 703–713

17. *Journal of the American Medical Association* (JAMA) (2004; 291:335–342).

18. *Practical Diabetes International* (2002; 19: 22–24)

Further References

•*Diabetes Care* 26 (January 1, 2003): 16–23. [The Strong Heart Study]

•Heart Protection Study Collaborative Group. "MRC/BHF Heart protection study of cholesterol lowering with simvastatin in 20,536 high-risk individuals: a randomized placebo-controlled study." *Lancet* 360, no. 9326 (July 6, 2002): 7–22.) [Heart Protection Study]

•UK Prospective Diabetes Study (UKPDS) Group 34. "Effect of intensive blood-glucose control with metformin on complications in overweight patients with type 2 diabetes." *Lancet* 352 (September 12, 1998): 854–865.

Appendix II
Quick Definitions Page

This is a not-so-quick Quick Definitions Page. This is also not a comprehensive list of medical terms. I have tried to pick out words in this book that may not be familiar to a non-medical person and define these terms in a comfortable doctor–patient conversational manner.

Glucose measurements

Glucose test can be done on whole blood or plasma.

Plasma is the liquid portion of blood after the red blood cells have been removed.

Glucose tests done in laboratories are usually done on plasma. These tests are the standard for accuracy.

Home glucose tests are done on whole blood, and home glucose meters use a formula to convert the readings to a plasma result. Older meters reported the results as a whole-blood result.

Some of us still say *blood sugar* or *blood glucose* when we should be saying *plasma glucose.* I may have made that mistake a few times in this book. If I did, you now know what I should have said. I have noticed that the test done on finger-stick blood may be a little higher than a laboratory test done at the same time. This is because the capillary blood drawn from your finger has a little higher glucose concentration than venous blood drawn from your forearm.

Glycohemoglobin or A1c
These terms are commonly used to describe a test that provides a look at your average glucose levels for the past two to three months. This test also serves as a marker of risk for future complications (*see* Chapter 7 for more details).

Lipid profile/lipid panel
This refers to a group of tests usually done at the same time that includes cholesterol, triglyceride, LDL, and HDL (*see* Chapter 7 for more details).

LDL cholesterol
We commonly associate this test with the risk of vascular disease such as heart attacks and strokes. Some people call it the "bad cholesterol." LDL (low density lipoprotein) is basically a transport system in the bloodstream for moving cholesterol, triglycerides, and other fats from the liver out to other tissues in the body, such as arteries.

HDL cholesterol
Higher levels of this are associated with lower risk of vascular disease. Sometimes known as the "good

cholesterol," HDL (high density lipoprotein) is also a transportation system that moves cholesterol, triglycerides, and other fats from body tissues back to the liver. Essentially, it is a cleaning system for the arteries.

Triglycerides
This is another form of fat circulating around in the blood. It is found stored in highly visible places around the body such as butts and bellies.

Cholesterol
Cholesterol is another fat seen on laboratory reports and is usually associated with the risk of vascular disease. However, cholesterol is not all bad. It has many other essential functions in the body. Cholesterol is an important constituent of cell walls and is the precursor of bile acids and many hormones, which include estradiol, testosterone, and cortisol.

Creatinine
Creatinine is a waste product of muscle metabolism that is filtered into urine by the kidneys. Increased creatinine levels in blood indicate kidney damage.

Albumin/creatinine ratio
(Alb./Creat Ratio) This test reflects the loss of small amounts of protein in the urine. A result above 30, confirmed by a repeat test, is an indicator of very early kidney damage (*see* Chapter 7).

Microalbuminuria – alb./creat. ratio >30 and <300 mcg/mg
Albuminuria – alb./creat. ratio >300 mcg/mg or urine albumin over 300 mg. per 24 hours

Statins

A common term for a large group of cholesterol-lowering drugs. Some common ones are: Zocor (simvastatin), Lipitor (atorvastatin), Mevacor (lovastatin), Lescol (fluvastatin), and Crestor (rosuvastatin).

Sulfonylureas

A group of medications that stimulate insulin-producing cells in the pancreas (beta cells) to produce more insulin. This class includes some of the first drugs to become available for the treatment of type 2 diabetes, such as Diabinase (chlorpropamide) and Orinase (tolbutamide). Newer drugs in this class include Glucatrol (glipizide); Micronase, Diabeta, Glynase (glyburide); and Amaryl (glimepiride). Side effects include weight gain and increased risk of hypoglycemia. I generally tried to avoid using these medications. If forced to choose one, it would be Amaryl.

Glucophage (metformin)

An excellent, inexpensive medication that enhances glucose uptake in muscle and reduces glucose production in the liver. This is a good first-line medication for type 2 diabetes.

Actos (pioglitazone)

Both of these medications reduce insulin resistance in muscle and fat tissue and reduce glucose production in the liver resulting in lower plasma glucose levels. My choice of these two is Actos because it is more effective in lowering triglycerides and raising HDL. Both of these medications can have the side effect of weight gain and/or edema.

Byetta (exenatide) and Victoza (liraglutide) are incretin mimetics. Januvia (sitigliptin) and Onglyza (saxagliptin) are DPP-4 inhibitors.
A little explanation is needed. Incretin hormones are released from our gut when we eat. These hormones have a significant effect on our blood glucose levels. They improve glucose stimulated insulin release from our Beta cells, regulate glucagon secretion, slow stomach emptying and preserve beta cell life. There is a progressive decline in the incretin hormones in type 2 diabetes. Incretin mimetics such as Byetta and Victoza replace one of these deficient hormones, GLP1 by injection. Medications such as Januvia and Onglyza inhibit an enzyme (DPP-4) that degrades the incretin hormones. These are exciting new medications that hold great promise for everyone with diabetes.

Byetta is one of my favorite medicines for people with type 2 diabetes. It comes in a prefilled pen and is given by subcutaneous injection before breakfast and dinner. Byetta has multiple effects such as improving insulin release, reducing glucagon secretion (which has the effect of reducing the liver's glucose production), slowing gastric emptying, and reducing appetite. It has a desirable side effect of weight loss. It can be added to my other favorite medication, Glucophage (metformin), if needed for better diabetes control.

Insulin preparations
My favorite insulins include Lantus (glargine), Humalog (lispro); and Novolog (aspart). Lantus insulin has a long duration of effectiveness (24 hours) with no peak. It provides a steady background insulin. For example, 24 units will provide 1 unit/hour for 24 hours with no significant peak. It can be given once daily and is adjusted to control the fasting glucose

level. NPH and Lente insulins last twelve to sixteen hours and require two injections daily to be effective, and both have a peak effect about six to eight hours after injection. This peak effect increases the risk of hypoglycemia. The peak effect problem of long-acting insulin becomes a benefit when we are discussing rapid-acting insulins such as Humalog and Novolog. The conversion of carbohydrates in one's diet into glucose in one's blood is rapid with a peak in blood glucose at about one hour after starting a meal. Humalog and Novolog insulin can be taken at the beginning of a meal and have a rapid onset of action; they will peak at about the same time as the glucose from the meal, at about one hour. This helps control the after-meal blood glucose rise. Regular insulin, on the other hand, has a slower onset of effect and peaks at about two hours, causing it to miss the peak blood glucose effect by about one hour. The result is higher after-meal blood glucose results.

Glucagon
Glucagon is a hormone secreted by the alpha cells in our pancreas. Glucagon is responisible for allowing the liver to release glucose when needed to maintain our blood glucose levels in the normal range. Unfortunately, Glucagon is released in inappropriate times in people with diabetes causing higher than expected blood glucose levels, seen commonly before breakfast.

Glucagon is available commercially as an injection for the emergency treatment of low blood glucose levels.

Goal Sheet

(Decide on your goals after discussion with your physician)

Test	Suggested Goal	Your Results	Your Goal
1. Home blood sugar test			
Before breakfast	90 to 130		
Before lunch	90 to 130		
Before dinner	90 to 130		
Before bedtime	100 to 140		
3:00 AM	90 to 130		
2. A1c hemoglobin	7		
3. Blood pressure (BP)	130/80		
4. Albumin/creatinine ratio	<30		
5. Cholesterol total	<200		
6. LDL cholesterol	<70		
7. HDL cholesterol			
In men	>40		
In women	>50		
8. Triglyceride	<150		
9. Abdominal girth			
For males	<40 inches		
For females	<35 inches		
10. Foot exam (yearly)			
11. Eye exam (yearly)			

Combined Diet, Exercise, and Blood Record

Date AM	3:00 AM	Before Breakfast	Before Lunch	Before Dinner	Bedtime
			PM		
	1 2 3 4 5 6 7 8 9 10 11 12 1 2 3 4 5 6 7 8 9 10 11 12				

David Calder, MD

Risk Factor Management Form Suggested form for tracking long-term factors					
Date					
BP					
A1c					
Alb/ creat. ratio					
Choles- terol					
LDL chol.					
HDL chol.					
Triglyc- eride					
Aspi- rin use yes/no					
Weight					
Waist size					
Foot exam (each year)					
Eye exam (each year)